THE POSTPARTUM HUSBAND

CONTENTS

COPING

COPING WITH SPECIFIC SITUATIONS

WHAT YOU MIGHT BE FEELING:

TREATMENT OPTIONS

MEDICATION

SUPPORT

SPECIAL CONSIDERATIONS

RECOVERY

To Bruce, my hero

Introduction:

WHY YOU SHOULD READ THIS BOOK

You might be reading this because your wife asked you to read it. Or, you might be reading this because you're really worried about what's going on at home.

Or, perhaps you're reading it. . . .

- *. . . Because you haven't had sex in three months and she doesn't seem to be bothered at all by this.*

- *. . . Because she's tired most of the time and hasn't been as available to you as much as you'd like and your marriage feels like it's too much work right now.*

- *. . . Because you think she has indulged in this bad mood thing for long enough and your patience is wearing thin.*

- *. . . Because you feel frustrated by her constant irritability and pessimistic outlook.*

- *. . . Because she is terrified about the way she feels and is looking for a way out.*

- *. . . Because you're quite exhausted yourself, and confused about what to do to make things better for both of you.*

You know things are not right at home. You've just had a baby. You, and everyone else, expected that life would be wonderful and full of joy. But it's not. Whatever your reason for picking up this book, let me reassure you with one point: You may not *want* to read this, but it *will* help you confront these issues. The problems at home need to be addressed. You know it. She knows it. So, here are some facts:

- Research has shown us that a woman's depression will improve markedly with the consistent support of a significant other.

- The longer you pretend that the depression will go away by itself and deny it is really happening, the longer her recovery will take.

- The more you expect of her, the greater your demands, the more difficult her recovery will be.

- The harder you are on yourself, the less resources you will have to carry you through each day.

- You have much more power to affect the outcome of how you both feel than you might think you do.

- Your wife *will* get better. Things will settle at home, in time. You will have your wife and your life back. But for now, it's important for you to take a look at some of the issues impacting your life right now.

It's important for her.
It's important for you.
It's important for your marriage.

IDENTIFYING THE PROBLEM:

ONE:

*"We just had a baby and now
our lives have turned upside down."*

UNDERSTANDING PPD

- Postpartum depression (PPD) affects 20–30% of all postpartum women. *(The term PPD will be used throughout the book to include all postpartum illnesses, such as postpartum obsessive-compulsive disorder, panic disorder, generalized anxiety and depression.)*

- PPD is a medical condition that can be treated successfully.

- PPD is a clinical depression that can occur any time immediately after birth up to a year postpartum.

- If your wife has been diagnosed with PPD, it's very important for you to be informed and part of the treatment. *(If you're not sure whether your wife has PPD, but one of you thinks something is wrong with the way she is feeling, it's time to have a doctor or mental health professional evaluate the situation. This book will help you understand PPD, but it does not take the place of a comprehensive evaluation and diagnosis.)*

- PPD can strike without warning—in women with no history of depression or women who have had it before. It can happen to women who are highly successful in their careers or women who stay home with their children. It can strike women in stable marriages and conflictual marriages, as well as single women, and adoptive mothers. It can happen to women who love their baby more than anything in the world. It can happen after the first baby, or after the fourth.

• It can happen to women who swore it would never happen to them.

• It is not completely understood why PPD affects some women and not others—why women who have many risk factors may not experience it, and others who have no risk factors may end up with a full blown episode.

• Women are twice as likely to experience depression than men.

• Women are most at risk to experience emotional illness following the birth of a baby than at any other time.

What is Depression?

• Our best explanation is that genetic, biological, psychological and environmental forces combine in such a way as to influence the development of depression. Though we may not know precisely what causes it, we do know that depression is associated with a biochemical imbalance in the brain.

• This biochemical imbalance can occur for several reasons:

  ✦ *Genetic predisposition*: Depression is known to run in families.

  ✦ *Previous history*: Previous episodes put your wife at greater risk for depression.

  ✦ *Physical, emotional or sexual abuse, alcoholic parent.*

 ✦ *Early childhood loss*; particularly death of parent.

 ✦ *Life stressors:* (change or loss of job, move to new
    home or city, recent illness (self or loved one),
    loss of loved one, divorce or separation (self or
    parents).

• Risk factors do not cause depression. They merely set the stage or
  create an opportunity for it.

Two:

"Everyone says this is the Baby Blues.
Is it?"

DIFFERENTIATING BETWEEN
BLUES AND DEPRESSION

- Baby blues are often confused with PPD. Baby blues typically begin on day three postpartum and usually last a few hours to a couple of weeks.

- Baby blues are not an illness. The blues are common (affecting 60–80% of postpartum women), the symptoms resolve spontaneously and require no professional intervention.

- Baby blues are primarily a result of the dramatic hormonal drop that occurs postpartum and can be influenced further by the discomfort brought on by childbirth and the stressors related to the transition from hospital to home to motherhood.

- Symptoms of baby blues are: moodiness, irritability, crying, feelings of frustration and inadequacy, intermittent anxiety, exhaustion.

- If your wife does not like the way she is feeling, well-meaning family or friends may try to reassure her by telling her it's just "the blues." It may or may not be.

- *However, If her symptoms last beyond two to three weeks postpartum,* it's time for a medical work-up and/or discussion with her doctor.

- During the first couple of postpartum weeks, try to make sure she:

  + Rests as much as possible

  + Gets help with household duties

  + Delegates responsibilities

  + Eats well

  + Gets out of the house for short periods of time

  + Accepts help from those who offer

  + Receives comfort and reassurance and is not judged for anything she is feeling

  + Knows she can talk about the way she's feeling.

Three:

*"Now she has a diagnosis.
I just don't buy it."*

MAKING SENSE OUT OF THIS

- PPD is a real illness.

- She is not making this up.

- This did not happen because she's a bad mother, or doesn't love her baby enough.

- It did not happen because she's having negative thoughts about herself or about you or about your baby.

- It did not happen because she is weak and not working hard enough to get better.

- She cannot "snap out of it."

- This is not fair. This is not what you expected. But if your wife has been diagnosed with PPD, it will take a while for her to recover. Recovery may take weeks to months.

- She will get better. She will return to her "normal" self. She will begin to experience pleasure again. This will not happen overnight.

- The more supportive you are of her treatment, the smoother her recovery will be.

FOUR:

"Why did this happen?"

IT'S NO ONE'S FAULT

- PPD is nobody's fault. It is not your wife's fault. It is not your fault.

- Try to reassure your wife that there is *nothing* she has done to make this happen.

- Often, when we are struck by something we do not understand, we try to cast blame on someone or something. This will be counterproductive.

- Remember that we do not know exactly why this happened. What we *do* know is what to do to maximize the healing process.

- Do not spend excessive energy trying to figure out what went wrong or why this happened. Your search for a reason will frustrate you and it will keep your wife spinning along side of you. Save your energy for navigating through this unfamiliar territory.

FIVE:

"How long will this last?"

GOING WITH THE FLOW

- PPD is different for every woman. The most important factor here is that your wife receives proper treatment.

- Trust you or your wife's instinct if something feels out of sync. If *either* one of you think something is wrong—it probably is.

- PPD can feel as though it will never end. Some husbands feel PPD steals their wife away and leaves behind a trail of anger, resentment and frustration. Her symptoms will resolve. She will feel better again.

- You will get your wife back.

- If your wife is in treatment, this usually means therapy and often, medication. With this regime, relief from the acute symptoms should take place within the 2–6 week framework given for most antidepressants to reach maximum effectiveness. Initial and immediate comfort should be obtained through a relationship with a good therapist.

- One of the most helpful things you can do to expedite this process is to help her feel understood and cared for. It's important for you to let this be known to her, whether or not you completely "believe" in this illness, understand it or the process of recovery. She needs to think you understand it and will be comforted by your words of support, if they are heartfelt, *even if* you remain skeptical about much of this. I'm all for going through the motions if it gets you through the haze, as long as you are doing it *without* judgment, sarcasm, or anger.

• What you do or do not do during this period, will impact your wife's recovery process.

• If this is especially difficult for you because you just don't get it, do it anyway. Get as much information and support along the way as you can so it all begins to make more sense.

SIX:

*"If she were really depressed,
she couldn't be faking it this well."*

THE POWER OF PRETENSE

• Postpartum women yearn for control over the unpredictability of
the current situation. Many are driven to exert control by
maintaining a strong outward appearance.

• If your wife is someone who likes to be in control (and who doesn't!),
and/or tends to be perfectionistic or compulsive in some ways,
it is likely that she will be terrific at perpetuating the illusion
that all is fine, particularly to the outside world.

• It is very important to her that she "looks good" on the surface.
Remember that just because she's able to go through the motions and continue to take care of things—this in no way di-
minishes her ongoing battle with the way she is feeling.

• Do not let the facade lull you into thinking she is feeling better
than she is. Check it out. Ask her.

• Remind her that you know how bad she feels, even if she isn't
telling you. This will validate her pain, which is more important than you might realize, and it will let her know you are
available if she needs you.

- Do not assume everything is okay because she says everything is okay.

SEVEN:

"She used to be so strong"

MISCONCEPTIONS ABOUT DEPRESSION

THESE BELIEFS ABOUT DEPRESSION ARE
NOT TRUE:

- *Women who are depressed cannot function.*

- *Women who are clinically depressed should always be in a hospital.*

- *Women who have PPD should not be left in charge of their baby's care.*

- *Women with PPD want to hurt their babies.*

- *If my wife were really depressed, she would never be able to go to work and do as well as she's doing.*

- *If my wife were strong, she would be able to get through this without professional help.*

- *If she takes medication for depression, she must be severely ill.*

- *If she is depressed, she might really go crazy.*

- *Depression is all in her head.*

EIGHT:

"Why is she so irritable all the time?"

SYMPTOMS OF PPD

If your wife has PPD she is most likely feeling:

- Irritable

- Weepy

- Sad

- Extremely anxious

- Scared

- Nervous

- Hopeless

- Exhausted

- Inadequate as mother and wife

- Disinterested in sex

- Unable to experience pleasure

- Worried about her negative, intrusive thoughts

- Confused

- Unable to concentrate

- Unable to sleep

- Unable to eat

- Worried she is going crazy

- Concerned this will never get better

- Afraid you will leave her

- Guilty or ashamed about how she is feeling

Some *physical* symptoms may include:

- Stomach problems/nausea

- Shortness of breath

- Headaches

- Lightheaded or feeling "unreal"

- Numbness/tingling

- Chills/hot flashes

- Trembling

- Palpitations

NINE:

*"Why is she asking the same things
over and over and over and over?"*

RUMINATING

- Ruminating refers to:
    - ✦ Repetitive thoughts

    - ✦ Thoughts that preoccupy the mind

    - ✦ Racing thoughts

    - ✦ Thoughts that monopolize or engross the mind
      beyond reason

    - ✦ Obsessive thoughts

- Your reassurance, though certainly encouraged, probably will
  have very little effect on her tendency to ruminate.

    - ✦ No matter how many times you tell her you are
      not getting tired of this, she will think that
      you are.

    - ✦ No matter how many times you tell her she's a
      good mother, she will doubt this.

✦ No matter how many times you tell her the baby will be fine with the baby-sitter, she will worry constantly until she gets home.

• Your persistence and support are essential here, but you also will be most challenged, especially when she asks the same things over and over again, and when you see your responses do not make a difference. This will lead to frustration, and possibly withdrawal if you're not careful. Watch for signs that you are pulling away from her.

• One way to deal with her ruminating is to identify it for your wife. Tell her what she's doing. Explain what ruminating is and how you understand this is a symptom. Tell her this plan: You will reassure her two times for any given worry. After the second time, you will say a "cue word" (one that you both have agreed on previously, a word that means something to both of you. Examples of some that couples have used are: "Bermuda", "Picasso", "Jacuzzi", or whatever.) When this word is spoken, it's a signal to break the cycle. It's along the same lines as her snapping a rubber band on her wrist, which some women will do, to remind them to "stop" ruminating. It's not an easy thing to do, but having some objective reminder helps.

• Another trick that is useful is to keep her mind occupied with busy work. What works best is brain work—jobs that assign the brain to focus on task-oriented skills such as: crossword puzzles, jigsaw puzzles, counting or math problems, paint-by-numbers (really!), arts & crafts, organizing a closet or anything else that keeps her focused on something "mindless." The ruminations tend to decrease if her mind is busy with trivial distraction.

- Try not to get discouraged as this can become quite wearisome. Do not ignore her ruminations. This will only increase her anxiety and feelings of isolation from you. Try to find a balance between indulging her worries and disregarding them completely.

TEN:

"Her thoughts are scaring me."

DEALING WITH
NEGATIVE, INTRUSIVE THOUGHTS

- Many women experience very negative, sometimes scary, intrusive thoughts. These thoughts seem to come and go with their own power, and feel very real.

- These thoughts are often fears that:

  - ✦ She will hurt herself

  - ✦ She will hurt her baby

  - ✦ Something catastrophic will happen beyond her control

  - ✦ Something by default will happen ("if I slip with this sharp knife in my hand, I could injure my baby.")

- Many women do *not* share the fact that they are experiencing these thoughts due to a fear that they will be misunderstood and risk being labeled crazy or unfit.

- Ask your wife if she's experiencing any negative, scary thoughts.

Reassure her that this is normal and that treatment will ease the burden of these thoughts.

• Try not to be afraid of these thoughts. Your fear will exacerbate her preoccupation with worry.

• These negative thoughts are common and are *not* an indication that she will harm her baby.

• If they persist, these thoughts respond well to medication.

• Let your wife know that you trust her. Remind her that these are just thoughts and they do not mean that she will take action on them.

• The best defense against these thoughts is:

Talk about them → get them out → distract from them

• Encourage her to express her concerns about these thoughts, reassure her that she is safe and that you are confident that nothing bad will happen, then, change the subject and help her mind become busy with something else.

• Shame is almost always attached to these thoughts. Do your best to help her understand that these thoughts are "symptoms" and eventually they will go away.

• These thoughts should not be confused with thoughts that accompany a psychotic disorder. Those thoughts are bizarre and delusional in nature—thoughts that indicate a loss of touch with reality. ("This child is not my baby. She is the devil and I need to relieve her from her pain to prevent evil doings . . .") Thoughts such as these require immediate, emergency intervention, usually hospitalization. *Contact her doctor immediately or take her to the closest emergency room if your wife is experiencing delusional thoughts or hallucinations.*

- If your wife is troubled by her thoughts, she has *not* lost touch. She is very much in touch, which is precisely why she is so troubled. Tell her you know it *feels* like she is losing her mind, but she is *not*.

ELEVEN:

"She never used to worry like this."

COPING WITH ANXIETY

- PPD is often an agitated depression. This means its predominant symptom often is excessive anxiety.

- Anxiety can take many forms. It can appear as worry, preoccupation with thoughts, preoccupation with physical health, obsessive thinking, panic attacks, sleeplessness, feelings of impending doom, nervousness.

- Physical manifestations are: palpitations, chest tightness, shortness of breath, stomach problems, nausea, weepiness, lightheadedness, fear of having a heart attack, shakiness, sensation of numbness.

- Anxiety can affect other areas of functioning:

  + It can affect sleep, often causing insomnia.

  + It can affect mood, often causing severe irritability.

  + It can affect ability to function, often creating new fears or phobias about being alone or about being with others.

✦ It can affect self-esteem.

• Anxiety is one of the leading reasons for the misdiagnosis of post-partum depression. Sometimes, doctors will treat only the anxiety symptoms, which may be pervasive, failing to recognize the larger picture. Most typical is the presence of a primary depression with secondary anxiety.

• Many first treatment choices for anxiety (anti-anxiety medications) will *not* treat an underlying depression.

• Antidepressants that are used to treat PPD *will* also treat the anxiety that accompanies it.

TWELVE:

*"I keep reassuring her,
but nothing helps."*

THE NATURE OF DEPRESSIVE THINKING

- When someone is depressed, they think negatively. When someone thinks negatively, it reinforces how depressed she feels.

- If you can think more positively, you will feel better. This is very hard to do when you're depressed.

- Some experts believe that the negative thoughts are *symptoms* of depression. Treat the depression, and you will begin to think less negatively. Others say that negative thoughts *cause* the depressive thought process. Learn to reframe the thinking into positive channels and you will begin to feel better, these experts believe.

- Then, there are some who believe that both viewpoints are true. Treat the depression, and you will reduce the negative thinking. While you are doing that, work on restructuring the thought process to integrate more positive thinking, thereby reinforcing healthy functioning.

- It doesn't really matter "how" she got this, whether it was negative thinking habits, or a biologic imbalance. *Either way*, the most effective treatment is the combination of antidepressant medication (to restore the neurotransmitter balance) and psychotherapy (to unlearn self-destructive thought patterns).

THIRTEEN:

"She's not sleeping. She's exhausted.
Could that be the problem?"

COPING WITH SLEEP DEPRIVATION

• Most new mothers will experience exhaustion and overwhelming fatigue during the first few months (less often, up to a year) after childbirth. Night after night of interrupted sleep will directly affect her moods throughout the day.

• Steps should be taken to try to augment her sleep as much as possible, particularly in the first few months postpartum.

• Try to distinguish between sleep difficulties that are a result of midnight awakenings or restless babies, from sleep difficulties that seem independent of the baby's activities. In other words, *is your wife sleeping okay as long as the baby is sleeping?*

• Sleep disturbances that persist in spite of your sleeping baby, need to be addressed with her doctor.

• Several nights in a row of little or no sleep (less than three hours), usually indicates the need for an evaluation by her healthcare provider.

• Sleep deprivation can have a dramatic impact on how a woman feels during the postpartum period. In some cases, women who are in acute distress discover that after a few nights of uninterrupted sleep, their other symptoms may subside.

• If your wife is suffering from sleep deprivation, make sure she lets her doctor know *precisely* how much or how little sleep she's actually getting. We often hear: "I can't remember the last time I had a good night's sleep." Or, "I haven't sleep in weeks!" Although these exaggerations are understandable, her doctor needs to know exactly how many hours of sleep she's getting to determine whether intervention is warranted.

FOURTEEN:

"Aren't we overreacting here?"

COMING TO TERMS

- Let's face it, this is the last thing you expected and certainly the last thing you feel like dealing with after having a baby.

- PPD can challenge even the most solid marriages. You cannot afford to take this lightly and hope it goes away on its own.

- Your wife needs a great deal from you right now. She is not making this up. If there's one thing I can guarantee, it's this: the more you resist, the longer this whole process will take.

- Resistance can take many forms. It can be denial, or withdrawal, or anger, or acting-out, attention-seeking behaviors. It can be passive uninvolvement or hostile confrontation. Or, in its most common state, it can be neutral disconnection. This is a way of disengaging from the crisis, simply by not addressing it. This does not mean you are not a wonderful partner who cares very much about the well being of your wife. But it may mean it's easier just to "not deal" with this. Remember, when left to travel by its own wind, the force of the crisis can blow the two of you astray, leading your marriage into unsteady territory.

- Do not surrender to the temptation to walk away from this.

COPING

FIFTEEN:

"Why is she saying these things?"

WHAT SHE MIGHT BE FEELING AND WHAT YOU CAN *DO ABOUT IT*

- *"She's crying all the time"*: This is a normal response and though it's difficult to witness, it is not an indicator of how serious her illness is. She may just need to cry and cry. Let her cry. Ask her, when she is *not* crying, what you can do to help when she feels like that. Some women like to be left alone. Others prefer to be held close. Ask her.

- *"She feels so guilty about everything"*: Of course she feels guilty. She feels like she's letting everyone down. After all, lots of women have babies and feel fine. Well, her guilt will definitely get in the way of her feeling better, so remind her that when she's feeling better she will no longer feel this way. Her guilt will feel as though it's based on reality, but in fact, it's based on faulty thinking, which will improve as she moves through recovery.

- *"She believes she's a bad mother"*: Tell her, simply, that she is a good mother. Point out the things she is doing, in spite of feeling so bad, that make her a good mother. Good mothers get sick, too. This has nothing to do with her ability to be a good mother. If she is unable to care for your child at this time, reassure her that the baby is receiving love and comfort from substitute caretakers and he or she will be fine.

- *"She says we should never have had this baby"*: She's feeling overwhelmed and the decision to have the baby is staring her right in the face. This, too, is largely based on distorted thinking, so it's best not to give it too much power by reinforcing it. Do not overreact. Simply let her say it and continue to tell her what a good job she's doing.

- *"She worries that I'm going to leave her"*: Remind her that you have no intention of going anywhere and that you are in it for the long haul. You may have to remind her on a regular basis.

- *"She's so irritable and difficult to live with sometimes"*: This is a hard one, because it's tough being around someone who feels so bad all the time. You need to build in breaks for yourself and try to remember not to take the things she says personally. She may lash out at you more often than usual because it feels safe for her to do so. This won't feel good, but try not to make it worse by reciprocating. Try to remain neutral, set limits, identify what's going on for her and remove yourself from the situation, if possible.

- *"She's afraid she might harm the baby"*: If she's saying she's afraid she might hurt your baby, try to assess whether *you* are worried about that also, or, if it's an extension of feeling inadequate and fearful. Most postpartum women worry that they may do something wrong or act in some way that may indirectly cause harm to the baby. This fear is common and almost always come from the anxiety that is so pervasive in PPD. Again, remind her she is doing everything fine, and you have confidence in her ability to mother your baby.

- *"She's can't stand to be alone"*: This is usually most problematic when her symptoms are acute, during the very early stages of treatment. If at all possible, it's helpful to have someone she feels comfortable with stay with her for a while. A support person at this time is needed to reduce her feelings of panic that she might associate with being alone with the baby. This can be you, or your mother, or a sister, friend, neighbor, childcare person, etc. Do not encourage her to be alone for long periods of time if it creates significant anxiety right now. This will get better as she begins to feel stronger and more secure in her new role as a mother.

- *"She seems preoccupied with physical complaints":* Anxiety and depression often manifest in physical ways, most commonly as: headaches, dizziness, diarrhea, shortness of breath, palpitations, lethargy, neck and upper back spasms, jaw pain (teeth grinding), numbness or tingling in arms and legs, hot flashes, chills, nausea. Extreme cases can involve vomiting, vision problems, and migraines. It's important to check out all physical complaints with a good examination by her general practitioner, including a thyroid screening. The thyroid screening is essential, because thyroid dysfunction is not unusual following childbirth and some of the symptoms mimic depression, so you want to rule that out.

- *"She thinks she is crazy:* PPD makes women feel like they are going crazy. They are not.

- *"She's fearful she will never get better":* She feels like she will always feels like this. This is not true, although it feels that way, for sure. You might have to tell her, repeatedly, that she will get better. The cloud that hangs over her is very difficult to see through. Help her through the fog by reminding her that there *is* a way out, it just takes longer than she would like to wait right now.

Sixteen:

"This is not the way I would be handling it."

WHAT WORKS FOR YOU . . .
MAY NOT WORK FOR HER

- Men respond differently to stress than women do.

- It is tempting for you to think about how YOU would react if you felt this way. You want to fix it. Make it go away. Find a reason. Find a solution.

- This won't work.

- Here are some generalizations, about men and women as examples:

Think about how you might respond if you felt incapacitated by feelings of helplessness and sadness:

You'd want to be alone → she wants you there all the time.

You wouldn't tell anyone → she needs to talk.

You'd get up and out and run yourself through this → she stays inside and can't get up and go.

You'd isolate yourself at work → she craves support and comfort from others.

You'd withdraw from your partner → she yearns to be close to you.

You'd turn your sadness into anger → she feels inadequate and worthless.

- Obviously, this won't apply to everyone, and is admittedly, based on stereotyped descriptions. But if any of these hold true for you, you might inadvertently project some of these expectations onto your wife.

SEVENTEEN:

*"I think I know what would help,
but she's not doing it."*

YOU CANNOT FIX THIS

• You cannot make this go away.

• You cannot fix this. No matter how hard you try or how much you love your wife.

• Recovery takes a very long time. You must be willing to wait this out with her.

• Practical things that will help are:

    ✦ Helping around the house

    ✦ Setting limits with friends and family

    ✦ Accompanying her to doctor's appointments

    ✦ Educating yourself about PPD, reading the books your wife gives you

    ✦ Writing down the concerns and questions you have and taking them to her doctor or therapist.

- **The single most important thing for you to do to help is to sit with her. Just be with her.** No TV, no kids, no dog, no bills, no newspaper. Just you and her. Let her know you're there.

- This isn't easy to do, especially with someone who seems so sad or so distant. Five minutes a day is a good place to start.

Eighteen:

*"I think if she would just relax,
she would start feeling better."*

WHY WHAT YOU THINK WILL HELP—MAY NOT HELP

- It's extremely frustrating to live with someone who's depressed, especially when you have a new baby and it seems like the house is crowded with things that need to get done right now.

- Do not tell her what to feel or what not to feel. Do not say: "You should be happy, our baby is so wonderful." Or, "Don't be scared, everything is fine."

- Instead, validate what she's feeling. " I know you feel like you're not a good mother, but our baby is doing so well, that it's clear to me you're doing so many wonderful things with him." Or, "I know you're scared, but we're doing everything we need to do to get you feeling better."

- Some of the things you think she should do right now to feel better, may not work.

- Some of the things that previously made her feel good, may feel like too much effort at this time.

- Make a list, together, of the things that may provide an outlet for her so you can both refer to it when she needs a break.

NINETEEN:

"Whatever I say, backfires."

WHAT TO SAY . . .

- Her moods and emotional vulnerability will get in the way of good communication for now.

- Here's what you're up against:

  - ✦ If you tell her you love her, *she won't believe you.*

  - ✦ If you tell her she's a good mother, *she'll think you're just saying that to make her feel better.*

  - ✦ If you tell her she's beautiful, *she'll assume you're lying.*

  - ✦ If you tell her not to worry about anything, *she'll think you have no idea how bad she feels.*

  - ✦ If you tell her you'll come home early to help her, *she'll feel guilty.*

  - ✦ If you tell her you have to work late, *she'll think you don't care.*

But you *can:*

- Tell her you know she feels terrible.

- Tell her she will get better.

- Tell her she is doing all the right things to get better (therapy, medication, etc.).

- Tell her she can still be a good mother and feel terrible.

- Tell her it's okay to make mistakes, she doesn't have to do every-thing perfectly.

- Tell her you know how hard she's working at this right now.

- Tell her to let you know what she needs you to do to help.

- Tell her you know she's doing the best she can.

- Tell her you love her.

- Tell her your baby will be fine.

TWENTY:

"I try to help around the house."

WHAT TO DO . . .

- Answer the phone. Take a message. Or put the answering machine on.

- Throw in a load of laundry.

- Order take-out for dinner.

- Call her from work to check in. Call her again if she's having a bad day.

- Ask her if there is anything you can do to help.

- Look her in the eyes when she talks to you.

- Encourage her to get as much rest as possible.

- Intervene so she can get some uninterrupted sleep.

- Try to find some "you and me" time with no other distractions.

- Call a friend and solicit support.

- Listen to her.

- Be patient.

TWENTY-ONE:

"I wish she would snap out of it."

WHAT NOT TO SAY

- Do *not* tell her she should get over this.

- Do *not* tell her you are tired of her feeling this way.

- Do *not* tell her this should be the happiest time of her life.

- Do *not* tell her you liked her better the way she was before.

- Do *not* tell her she'll snap out of this.

- Do *not* tell her she would feel better *if only*: she were working, she were not working, she got out of the house more, stayed home more, etc.

- Do *not* tell her she should lose weight, color her hair, buy new clothes, etc.

- Do *not* tell her all new mothers feel this way.

- Do *not* tell her this is just a phase.

- Do *not* tell her if she wanted a baby, this is what she has to go through.

- Do *not* tell her you know she's strong enough to get through this on her own and she doesn't need help.

TWENTY-TWO:

"Should she stop breastfeeding?"

MAKE IMPORTANT DECISIONS AS A COUPLE/BREASTFEEDING

- In general, try to postpone any important decision until *after* she is feeling better.

- Decisions that cannot wait should be made together, whenever possible.

- Decisions about childcare, work, breastfeeding, etc. will feel enormous to her now. Help her sort this out by discussing the pros and cons of each decision.

- Do not underestimate how important her decision to continue breastfeeding is—no matter how badly she is feeling.

- For some women, breastfeeding may represent the most significant attachment at this time:

  ✦ It is often the primary source of gratification

  ✦ It may represent her only (perceived) success at this time

✦ It is something *she* can do, and no one else, reinforcing a feeling of value and importance

✦ It may compensate for any worries that she is
failing to attach to her baby.

- On the other hand, breastfeeding can *increase* stress under the
following conditions:

  ✦ If she experiences any physical problems related
  to breastfeeding such as sore nipples, breast
  infections, or difficulty with baby latching on.

  ✦ If your wife feels tied down or trapped in any
  way by the nursing relationship or demands
  of feeding.

  ✦ If she feels she is missing the opportunity for
  relief, i.e., someone else being able to feed
  baby while she is free to sleep, get out of the
  house, etc.

- Some women feel *better* when they discontinue breastfeeding due
  to the hormonal changes.

- Some women feel *worse* when they discontinue breastfeeding due
  to the hormonal changes.

- Any woman considering weaning, particularly if she is suffers
  with symptoms of PPD, must taper the feedings **very slowly**.

- This decision to discontinue breastfeeding should be made among
  you, your wife, you, your wife's doctor and your baby's doctor. The decision to stop breastfeeding is never an easy one.
  But remember this, no matter what, your baby will be fine.

Your baby will adjust whether he's being breastfed or bottlefed. Our consideration now is to maximize Mom's adjustment and sense of well-being. Everything else will follow.

- *If she's considering medication while breastfeeding,* this should be discussed with the doctor treating her, as well as your baby's pediatrician.

- There *are* medications that have been determined compatible with breastfeeding.

- This is always a risk-benefit analysis, weighing the risks of medications against the risks of an untreated illness.

* For more on breastfeeding and medication, see chapter (50)

TWENTY-THREE:

*"All of a sudden,
she doesn't want to do anything or go anywhere"*

EMOTIONAL PARALYSIS

- Remember she is scared, so she *feels* as if she's not able do anything, even if she is.

- Depression is a very self-absorbing illness. It feels like *everything* revolves around the way you are feeling.

- Try to help your wife find a balance between doing too much and not doing enough.

- Everything feels like it's too much. Her first response to doing anything is likely to be, "I can't." Or, "I don't feel like it." Or, "I'm not up to it."

- The most effective way to get her involved, even on a small scale, is to *acknowledge that you know how hard this is for her and always give her an option out*, just in case.

- For example:

Instead of: "C'mon, let's just go. If we wait for you to feel better, we'll never to anything . . . it will be fine."

Try this: "I know you don't feel like going, but it will be okay. Let's go for a little while. If you feel bad while we're there, we'll leave early and go home."

• Try to keep your expectations realistic.

TWENTY-FOUR:

"I think if she gets out, she'll feel better."

WHEN TO PUSH THE BOUNDARIES

- Here, I refer to "pushing" as encouraging beyond her instinctive resistance—helping her move beyond the temptation to remain inert.

- Do not make the mistake of thinking she can just decide not to feel this way. I know there are people, including many professionals, who will claim that positive thinking will provide the opposite force needed to get her moving in the right direction.

- This is true, in certain situations, at the right time. But if you prematurely expect her to "think" herself through this before she feels ready, she will retreat into her "he-doesn't-understand-how-I-feel" mode.

- Cognitive interventions (based on the concept that the way we think, affects the way we feel and if we can replace the negative thoughts with positive ones, we will feel better) are most effective in recovery phases. While symptoms are acute, however, it may be less effective.

- Since she is likely to interpret most things as negative right now, cognitive work should, in time, be an integral part of her recovery work.

- In the meantime, be careful how you respond to her negative thinking. It is very automatic for her and she does not believe she will ever be able to change the way she is thinking. She will.

- If you don't do this "right", it can backfire: The more she *feels* attacked, the further back she will go. "Pushing" must be done with love, support, and most important, some understanding of how hard this is for her.

- Determine when it's appropriate and even necessary to push and when it is not. For instance, she needs to push herself to get up, get dressed, and take care of the children, *no matter how bad she is feeling*. She does *not* have to push herself to go to a party with 200 people she doesn't know.

- In some instances, feeling depressed feels "easier" than finding the energy to get better. (This is when therapy can help.)

- Take her hand. Take it slow.

TWENTY-FIVE:

"She's doing too much."

SET LIMITS

- For some women, their need to keep "doing" outweighs the fact that they don't feel like doing anything.

- Keeping busy feels as if it can distract them, however momentarily, from the grip of the illness.

- Remember to make sure she is resting, eating well, and taking care of her physical self.

- Signs that your wife might be overdoing it:

  ✦ She cannot say no

  ✦ She is repeatedly doing things for others at the expense of her rest or time to herself

  ✦ She is not able to give herself permission to do what *she* wants to do

  ✦ She is constantly irritable, frustrated, tired, angry, blaming others for how bad she feels.

- If your wife is doing too much, help her by making it easier for her *not* to do some of those things. Remind her how important it is for her to take care of herself. Keeping busy is good. Overextending herself is not.

TWENTY-SIX:

"She's not doing enough."

ENCOURAGE, DON'T PRESSURE

- Keep things simple. Keep plans manageable.

- Try to remember that her inactivity is directly related to her illness. As she feels better, she will slowly resume normal activities.

- Help her resist the temptation to surrender to what "seems" to be the most desirable alternative—not doing anything.

- It's hard for others to understand how profoundly difficult it is to do *anything*, when you feel this way.

- Be careful not to judge or express your anger. Your disappointment is normal.

- *If your wife is not functioning, that is, she is not able to get up and do the minimum, such as get dressed, take care of the children, etc., you must seek professional help.*

COPING WITH SPECIFIC SITUATIONS

"What do I do If..."

TWENTY-SEVEN:

"She's having an anxiety attack."

HOLD STEADY

• Once you have determined (through a medical evaluation and therapeutic diagnosis) that she is experiencing anxiety attacks—try to keeps these points in mind:

• It "feels" like things are out of control, even when they are not.

• Your wife needs grounding during an attack, whether it's at 11:00 at night or 3:00 in the morning. That means she needs to feel that she is safe and her thoughts are in check. Speak directly to her fear and offer reassurance.

• Her thoughts are distorted right now. Even though they do not make sense to you, they make total sense to her. And they are her reality right now.

• Clarify where things stand. Tell her what is going on.

• Oversimplify things for her. Keep everything manageable.

• Look her in the eyes.

• Touch her. Even if this feels bad to her, which it might. Let her know you are there. Hold her hand. Touch her back. Whatever feels most comfortable to you and least threatening to her.

• Tell her even though this feels terrible, *nothing bad is happening*. It just *feels* bad.

• She is not having a heart attack. She is not dying. She is not going crazy. Remind her, gently.

• Anxiety attacks do pass. No matter how bad they feel. Waiting them out is essential. If you run to the emergency room every time she has an anxiety attack, you will be reinforcing her greatest fear that she is out of control and that you are fearful of this.

• Anxiety attacks respond well to cognitive therapy, supportive therapy and/or medication.

TWENTY-EIGHT:

*"She makes demands on my time or schedule.
I can't always be there when she wants me to."*

COMPROMISE

• Try to determine whether or not it is an emergency. Obviously, if you are frightened by what you hear, you need to respond appropriately.

• If you think her need for you to be with her is coming from fear of being alone during this time:

> ✦ Help her mobilize a support network of family and friends, who can be there on a regular basis.

> ✦ Let her know you would like to be there for her, but you are constrained by work, etc., and tell her the ways she can check in with you each day.

> ✦ Encourage her to develop a plan for each day, something that feels good and will keep her busy.

• Most likely she is feeling very guilty about "needing" you so much, particularly if she is not, by nature, a needy person.

Tell her you understand that this is part of the illness and that *this*, too, will get better as *she* gets better.

• Remember the paradox of this dilemma: If you run home to rescue her every time she asks for it, you will reinforce her belief that she cannot do this without you.

• Do not misinterpret her feelings of rejection or as an indication that you are doing the wrong thing.

• Offer positive reinforcement for each small effort she accomplishes on her own.

TWENTY-NINE:

"She doesn't want me to go to work."

MOVING FORWARD

- Chances are, your wife will resent the fact that you are going to work and your schedule "hasn't changed much."

- She is afraid her symptoms will get worse while you are away.

- Her symptoms *may* indeed get worse while you're away.

- She may respond to your going to work with anger or fear or worry or panic or despair.

- Try to set up some reasonable compromise between what she feels she needs from you right now in terms of your time and what you can realistically offer. Perhaps some short-term arrangement that would allow you to come home early a couple of days a week, for example.

- Her fear of being without you will subside as her symptoms are treated and as she gains confidence in her ability to care for your baby.

- Call and check in several times during the day if this would reassure to your wife.

THIRTY:

"She says she can't take this pain anymore."

LISTEN TO HER

- If your wife tells you she cannot take this pain anymore, it's a very serious statement that means it's time for an evaluation by someone who specializes in the treatment of depression.

- Remember, her thoughts are distorted and it is possible that things feel much worse to her than they appear to you.

- It is not up to you to determine whether she's at risk for hurting herself or someone else. A professional should determine it. Thoughts of hurting herself may be expressed in passive terms: "I don't want to die, I just want to get rid of this pain." *This is still a sign that she should seek professional help.*

- Stay with her. Ask her if she feels safe from harm. Help her make an appointment with someone she feels can help her. Call her doctor.

- Do not leave her alone.

THIRTY-ONE:

"She's blaming me for how she feels."

DON'T OVERREACT

- Her sadness and depression may manifest in anger and rage.

- There is a normal tendency to want to place blame on someone or something in an effort to make sense out of all of this.

- Do your best not to overreact to this.

- Do not take this personally.

- This does not mean you should accept abusive or hurtful behavior.

- Help her redirect her anger where it belongs, onto the illness, not you—and help her find constructive ways to release it.

THIRTY-TWO:

"She doesn't believe my words of reassurance."

UNDERSTANDING
HER LOSS OF CONFIDENCE

• Do you find yourself saying the same things over and over again? And she still doesn't believe you?

   ✦ About getting better?

   ✦ About you loving her?

   ✦ About not feeling guilty?

   ✦ About being a good mother?

   ✦ About the marriage being in trouble?

   ✦ About driving you crazy?

• Her feelings of self-doubt and inadequacy go way beyond her trust and confidence in your words right now.

• Her loss of confidence is directly related to her symptoms. That is, as her treatment progresses and she gains symptom relief, she will begin to feel more self-assured and secure about her feelings and decisions.

- Until then, continue to state what she needs to hear, even if you're afraid it means little to her now. It's important that she hears it.

- Take an index card. Write down a number of reassuring statements. Examples:

  - ✦ "I love you."

  - ✦ "You will get better."

  - ✦ "I am not going anywhere. I'm here for the long haul. I will always be here with you."

  - ✦ "I know you are doing the best you can. You are still strong. You have an illness that is making you feel bad. We are doing what we are supposed to be doing to get you better."

- Give this card to her and tell her to keep it with her always. Tell her to read it aloud and to herself, whenever she is worried about you or the relationship.

WHAT YOU MIGHT BE FEELING:

And what you can do about it

THIRTY-THREE:

YOU ARE TIRED

- You bet you are. New baby. Long hours. Interrupted sleep. Demands at work. Wife who is not feeling well and about whom you're quite worried and preoccupied . . .

- You need your sleep. Make sure you are doing what you need to do to ensure this. If you are forced to endure night after sleepless night due to baby's schedule or your wife's particular symptoms, you must compensate somehow, by resting when you can.

- The same goes for you, as it does for your wife, when it comes to maintaining your physical health by eating well, exercising, resting, etc.

THIRTY-FOUR:

YOU ARE WORRIED

• Of course you're worried. If you've seen this before, you know how devastating depression can be to a family. If you've never seen this before, you are finding that out now.

• Some of the things you might be worried about are:

  ✦ Your wife's well-being

  ✦ Your baby's well-being

  ✦ Your ability to endure this

  ✦ Finances

  ✦ What others are saying or thinking about all of this

  ✦ Will this ever go away?

  ✦ How you can help her

  ✦ How you can get out of this

- Get information. Get answers. Read. Talk to her doctors. Become involved in her treatment.

- The more out of the loop you are, the more misinformed and worried you will be.

- Talk to other husbands who have been through this. I know this one is hard, but finding out that you're not alone with this can be very healing and reassuring.

THIRTY-FIVE

YOU ARE FRUSTRATED

• It's understandable that you would feel extremely frustrated. You miss the way your wife used to be. This can put a strain on the relationship.

• Try to keep your frustration in line with the situation at the moment. Frustrations will build and build and often get dumped in the wrong place at the wrong time. Be aware of this tendency.

• Keep an eye on your reactions. If you think your feelings or actions are getting out of hand, you have a responsibility to yourself, your wife and your family, to take care of this.

• Do a quick inventory:

  ✦ What are your usual coping behaviors?

  ✦ Are they constructive? (Example: exercise, talking with friends, doing a project)

  ✦ Are they destructive? (Example: rage, drinking, withdrawal)

+ Are you okay with the way you are reacting to the stress of the current situation?

+ Has anyone mentioned they are worried about YOU?

+ Do you have a source of support that you could be tapping into? (Friend, therapist, parent, colleague)

THIRTY-SIX:

YOU ARE ANGRY

- No kidding. Of course you're angry.

- If you *don't* think you're angry about this situation, you're probably very good at pretending that you're not.

- This is a terrible situation you are living with. It is NOT what you had in mind when the two of you sat down and fantasized about having a baby.

- Anger is a normal, healthy response to this situation.

- Your anger must be channeled and expressed appropriately, so it doesn't make things worse.

- If anger has been a problem for you previously, please be honest with yourself about this and take steps to get support. Anger left out of control will become a danger to your relationship at this time.

- Remind yourself that you are angry at the situation and/or the illness, rather than your wife.

THIRTY-SEVEN:

YOU ARE CONFUSED

- It feels like you've lost your wife.

- She will be back.

- I imagine you do not like to feel out of control and this is one of those times when you are faced with a situation that leaves you feeling totally out of control.

- Again, you need information about the symptoms, course of illness, treatment, etc. Part of your confusion results from the uncertain nature of the illness.

- The more information you get, the more validation you will have about some of the things that feel so unclear.

THIRTY-EIGHT:

YOU ARE RESENTFUL

- Well, this won't get you anywhere, but it's certainly understandable. That's what happens when you believe all those people who told you this was going to be the best time of your life!

- Doctors, friends, family, childbirth classes—they don't tell you a lot about postpartum illnesses. Unfortunately, this sets up the family for a tremendous letdown and leaves everyone thinking they are the only ones who have ever felt this way.

- So the resentment is huge. It moves from resenting your wife for "putting you through this" all the way to the medical community and society at large, for making you feel like there's something wrong with your family.

- There is nothing wrong with your family. You have been blindsided by this illness and now need to regroup and get back on track.

THIRTY-NINE:

YOU ARE SCARED

- You might be afraid she might never get better. Or perhaps you're afraid she might really go crazy. You might wonder if you'll ever get your wife back.

- Most likely, all of this is new to you and that can be very unsettling. Admitting that you're scared is not easy, nor is it necessary, but understanding that this is part of why you are so worried or so frustrated or so angry—is important.

- Arm yourself with facts from the medical community and surround yourself with people who can provide practical and emotional support.

- Treat yourself, when possible, to activities or pleasures that relieve your tension.

FORTY:

YOU ARE EMBARRASSED/ASHAMED

- The stigma attached to emotional illness still exists. You might not be comfortable sharing the intimate details of your current struggles with just anybody.

- Pick and choose from the important people in your life, and decide with whom you can share your private concerns.

- This is more important than you might think, because holding back can create a "secret" that becomes quite burdensome to you and can actually increase your shame, by reinforcing it.

- You probably will find enormous relief in sharing some of what's going on with someone you trust.

FORTY-ONE:

YOU ARE FEELING MISUNDERSTOOD

- Things don't make sense right now.

- You do not understand why your wife is feeling what she is feeling or why she responds to you the way she does.

- You try your best to do everything right and she still feels terrible.

- You try as hard as you can to keep the house together, take care of the kids, say the right things, and still—things aren't getting better.

- You are in the unenviable position of having the heavy burden of her illness cast upon you with no instructions for a way out.

- The way out is to ride out the rough waves and make sure your wife receives proper treatment.

- Taking care of yourself and paying attention to her illness are the two most important things you can do right now.

Treatment Options

FORTY-TWO:

"We can get through this on our own."

GUIDELINES FOR SEEKING HELP

- If your wife is struggling with depression, and you think you both can get through this easily, without professional help, you are probably mistaken.

- If you think getting professional help means one of you or both are weak, get over it. There's way too much going on right now for you to allow misguided stereotypes we all grew up with, to interfere with your wife getting the help she needs.

- Time parameters vary, but if you notice things are not getting better, or getting worse, it's a good indication that help is needed.

- If *she says it's time to get help*—yet you feel you have no other indications—it's time to believe her and get help.

- How you feel about the value of therapy, psychiatrists, therapists, emotional illness, etc., is *almost* irrelevant. I say almost, because, of course it enters into this picture and will affect how you perceive what's going on. But unless you decide right now to give that up and proceed with finding good, professional help, recovery will take longer. I can almost guarantee that.

• What you want is a good psychiatrist, psychologist, social worker or other therapist who specializes in the treatment of depression and/or women's issues.

• Ask for a referral from her doctor or midwife, her doctor, or a close friend. A personal referral from someone you both trust, increases the likelihood that you will match well with this person. That doesn't mean that finding a name out of the phone book will lead you astray. In fact, I would suggest you do that, if you don't have any other sources of referral.

• Other places to go for referrals are:

  ✦ Many local hospitals have Women Centers now and have access to private practitioners who they refer to and trust.

  ✦ If your wife is breastfeeding, ask her to check out a breastfeeding support group in your area. They are wonderful sources of support and often are well-connected to professionals in the area.

  ✦ Search the Internet. There are many websites dedicated to the treatment of depression in general and others that are specifically geared toward postpartum illnesses. Check parenting and baby-related sites, then search for postpartum articles or message boards.

FORTY-THREE:

"How do I know if her doctor/therapist is good?"
(And worth all that money?)

THINGS YOU SHOULD KNOW
ABOUT HER TREATMENT

• Good therapy can be expensive. But expensive therapy isn't always good.

• Getting help for your wife has to be the priority here. If you are more worried about how much it costs, she will stay sick longer.

• When I speak to a woman on the phone, and she hesitates to come in for a consultation because she's worried about the cost, I ask her: If your baby were sick, would you hesitate to take him to the doctor? If your husband were bleeding profusely, would you hesitate?

• Her illness is real. She needs treatment.

• So, how do you know if her therapist or doctor is good? Ask yourself these questions:

  ✦ Did you feel comfortable with this person? (Yes, you should attend a session).

+ Does your wife like him/her? (This is more important than you might think. Connecting
with this person is half the battle)

+ How does your wife feel about her sessions? Does
she think it's helping? Does she feel good about
going? Does she trust this person and feel comfortable talking?

+ Try to find someone who works short-term and
focuses on the here-and-now, rather than issues from the past. These issues are important, but not necessarily productive at the
outset, when we want to manage symptoms.

• The cost of treatment is a very real concern. But so is her staying
sick, isn't it? Please do not let the financial issues get in the
way of her getting the help she needs. There are options. Slid-
ing scales. Insurance plans. Payment schedules. Bringing up
your worries about the money can actually sabotage her recovery by making her feel guilty. Be careful how you do that.

• Encourage your wife to discuss any financial concerns with her
therapist. Contact your insurance company. Depending on
your particular plan, find out whether you need a referral from
your primary and if so, try to find a therapist who is a provider
for your network. If not, find out whether or not they reim-
burse this particular therapist. Most insurance companies will
ask you the therapist's credentials to determine reimburse-
ment. If the therapist is not covered at all, find out what arrangement can be made.

FORTY-FOUR:

"Should I go to therapy with her?"

JOIN THE SESSION

- Yes, you should go to a session with her. Some women like their husbands to join them for the first one. Others prefer their husbands wait until a relationship has been established with the therapist. Ask your wife if she'd like you to go with her and when. Then do it.

- You are going for a few reasons:

    + To show your support

    + To meet her therapist and see who's "taking care" of her

    + To ask questions, to get information, to receive support

    + To provide information to the therapist about your wife, your relationship, relevant history, etc.

- PPD becomes a family issue. Do not let your wife carry the load of this illness alone. *Supporting her decision to go to therapy is vital for her recovery.* Remember, therapy for PPD should be short-term. In therapy terms, this usually means 3–5 months.

But she should receive initial relief right away. Depending on the severity of her illness, she should start feeling somewhat better in the first few weeks.

FORTY-FIVE:

"Our marriage feels strained."

IMPACT ON YOU AS A COUPLE

- Chances are good that you've either been walking around on eggshells or feeling like a time bomb for a while now.

- Depression will strain any marriage.

- Paradoxically, it's often the stronger marriages that get affected the most. This sometimes occurs because the partners feel confident that they can afford to put the relationship "on hold" during the crisis, while there is so much else to contend with.

- This can leave both feeling depleted, unloved, and alone.

- If you are worried about your marriage, take a close look at it.

- If you are not worried about your marriage, take a close look, anyway.

- There will be times when you feel as though *you* are doing all of the work holding the family together. Maybe you are.

- Your marriage can endure this crisis, no matter how bad it feels sometimes.

FORTY-SIX:

"She said she would rather die than feel like this."

SUICIDAL THOUGHTS

- Suicidal thoughts may be passive ("I would do anything to make this pain go away" or active ("I'm afraid I might really do something to hurt myself").

- Suicidal thoughts are to be taken very seriously.

- If your wife is having suicidal thoughts, she should be under the care of a physician who can prescribe antidepressants for relief.

- While she is in crisis, if she is having active thoughts of hurting herself, she should not be alone. Not at all. Sometimes, hospitalization may be necessary, but this is less likely if there is a strong support network of family or friends who can provide 24 hour watch for a while.

- Remember, thoughts of suicide are a symptom of severe depression. This may not be characteristic of your wife and can create a false sense of security. This means, for example, she may actually believe her distorted thought that you and your baby would be better off without her here. She may actually find comfort when she thinks of ending her life if she is tortured by the belief that her illness is a problem for the family and her pain is too much to bear. She is not thinking clearly right now. *Do what you have to do to protect her.*

- In severe cases, medications, sharp objects, weapons, should not be accessible to her.

- If you are worried about her well-being and cannot reach her doctor, go with her to an emergency room.

FORTY-SEVEN:

"We have everything under control."

EMERGENCY SITUATIONS

- These situations are rare, but warrant immediate intervention:
  - ✦ Talk of hurting herself

  - ✦ Bizarre thinking patterns, hallucinations, delusions

  - ✦ No sleep in several days. This means NO sleep, usually coupled with manic-like symptoms. Sleep deprivation can worsen symptoms

  - ✦ Noticeable withdrawal from all social contact

  - ✦ Preoccupation with death, morbid ideas, or religious ideation

  - ✦ Persistent feelings of despair and hopelessness

  - ✦ Expressions such as: "My children would be better off without me here."

- Emergency situations mean you should take her to the closest hospital, call 911, or arrange for childcare alternatives.

- **DO NOT LEAVE HER ALONE FOR ANY REASON.**

MEDICATION

*(I will not be discussing specific medications. There are a
number of good medications that are used to treat depression.
Specifics should be handled between you, your wife and her
doctor.)*

FORTY-EIGHT:

"I don't want her popping pills to get better."

UNDERSTANDING MEDICATION

• The decision to take medication is very complicated for you and your wife.

• You may not want your wife to be on medication.

• If you don't like the idea of medication, think about why not. Think about whether you want her to get better.

• Medication for depression is not a cop-out. It is medicine that is successfully used to treat a very real illness.

• Medication will not make her zombie-like or spaced out. It should, in fact, help her think more clearly and become more focused.

• Get as much information as you can. Ask questions. Find answers.

• Listen to her. If she thinks medication will be helpful and this has been recommended by a healthcare professional, it is usually best to defer to her judgment.

• If you are worried about what other people might think, don't tell anyone, or forget it. It's no one's business. If others judge you, your wife or the situation, they are misinformed.

- Medication, in combination with supportive therapy, has been shown to be the most efficient, effective treatment for clinical depression.

FORTY-NINE:

"How do I know what medication is best?"

OPTIONS

- Most often, antidepressants are used to treat PPD when it is moderate to severe. Doctors often prescribe SSRI antidepressants, Selective Serotonin Reuptake Inhibitors, because they are easily tolerated and have a high success rate.

- Medication may be indicated when symptoms:

  + Interfere with daily functioning

  + Become worrisome to you or your wife

  + Affect how she is sleeping and/or eating

  + Cause abrupt mood changes

  + Cause difficulty concentrating

  + Cause severe agitation or panic

  + Lead to suicidal thoughts.

- If the depression is associated with anxiety, many times your wife will be given anti-anxiety medication to take as needed, *par-*

ticularly while she is waiting for the antidepressant to take effect.
Anti-anxiety medications are potentially addictive, so if she
needs them on a regular basis, it's important that she taper
down before she stops. If she's taking them intermittently, or
"as needed", then tapering is less necessary. This should always be discussed with her doctor.

• She may also need something to help her sleep, if sleeplessness is
  a problem.

• Antidepressants can take anywhere from one week to as many as
  eight weeks to take full effect. This can be a difficult time to
  wait out for both of you. Remind her it takes time for these
  medications to work. For most SSRIs, it can take 2–6 weeks to
  reach maximum effectiveness.

• Antidepressants are *not* addictive.

• Her doctor is the best judge of what she should be taking. Be
  certain to address any and all concerns you have with the
  doctor.

FIFTY:

"She's still breastfeeding. Can she take medication?"

NURSING AND MEDICATION

• There are medications that are compatible with breastfeeding.

• This decision is a very personal and important one—one that should be made among you, your wife, your wife's doctor and your baby's doctor.

• Expert opinions vary on the "safety" of nursing and medication. It is always a risk-benefit analysis, weighing the risks of taking the medication against the risk of not treating the illness. Be sure you are clear about your doctor's position and make sure you are both in agreement with that position.

• Sometimes, a woman will put the needs of her baby before her own needs. This can be potentially serious if it interferes with proper treatment.

• The older your baby is, the less risk there is of exposure to the medication.

• Take the time to discuss this with your wife at length. The breastfeeding relationship is closely tied into her feelings of accomplishment and confidence as a mother right now. Listen carefully as she reveals what this relationship means to her right now, so you can help guide her.

• The very best thing your wife can do for her baby is to take care of *herself.* If medication becomes an issue for your wife, help her understand that her health is of paramount importance and your baby will be fine, whether breastfeeding continues or whether she has to stop.

• Believe it or not, your support of this process and any decision she may have to make is as important as the ultimate decision. Help her walk through this process.

Fifty-one:

"Will the drugs make her totally out of it?"

LIVING WITH SIDE-EFFECTS

- The side effects will vary from woman to woman and from medication to medication.

- Most of the unpleasant side effects, if there are any, will surface soon after beginning the medication, and usually will subside after a couple of weeks.

- Common side-effects of SSRIs are: agitation, nausea, difficulty sleeping, diminished sexual drive, headache, feeling jittery.

- Many women do *not* experience troublesome side-effects.

- If you or your wife notices anything unusual or bothersome after starting a new medication, check with your doctor.

- Side effects usually are not troublesome enough to warrant switching medications, and, if she can tolerate them, the side effects should diminish. However, if she can't tolerate them, there are many other medications she can try.

- Remind your wife to alert her doctor if she is taking any over-the-counter remedies, particularly if she is taking any herbal supplements.

- One of the most troublesome side effects of the newer antidepressants is a loss of sexual function. This can be a lack of desire, or difficulty achieving orgasm.

- If this side effect becomes a problem for your wife, encourage her to talk to her doctor about it, as there are options, such as changing the dose, switching to another medication, adding another medication.

- If this side effect becomes a problem for *you,* we'll discuss it next.

FIFTY-TWO:

"We have no sex life"

THE IMPACT ON SEXUAL FUNCTIONING

• This is common.

• This can be due to the depression or the treatment (as noted previously, antidepressants can negatively affect her sex drive).

• It is very important that you do your best to be patient and supportive.

• She knows only too well how disappointed you are. Try not to remind her.

• Remember, she is feeling tired, insecure, unattractive, unsure of herself, and rather undesirable.

• She needs to know she is loved, but sex may be out of the picture for her right now.

• Try to retain a sense of humor. The more of a problem you make of this, the more likely she is to retreat even further. It's frustrating, to be sure. Remember this is not about you. It's about how she's feeling in response to her illness and her treatment. It will not always be this way.

- Talk with her about alternative ways to maintain closeness. What feels good to her? What doesn't feel good right now?

- Check out the specifics: Can we hold hands? Can we snuggle on the couch? Can we kiss?

- Keep in mind that part of her fear may be this: *if the two of you engage in any physical contact, she may worry about arousing you and then letting you down. Because of this, she may avoid all physical contact.*

- If this is not the way you want it to be, let her know that you can tolerate the physical closeness without pressuring her for more sexual contact.

- Stay close. Hold her when you can. Let her know you can bear this. Your sexual relationship will resume as she gets symptom relief.

FIFTY-THREE:

"How long will she have to take medication?"

COURSE OF TREATMENT

- The American Psychiatric Association recommends staying on the antidepressant for 6–9 months after she starts feeling better.

- Her medication needs to be taken on a regular basis, according to her doctor's instructions.

- She should *not* discontinue the medication on her own when she starts feeling better. It is a temptation for many women and unfortunately, it increases the risk of relapse.

- Feeling better does *not* necessarily mean she should be off the medication. It may mean she is feeling better *because* she's taking it.

- If she relapses, the symptoms are likely to be worse and more difficult to treat.

- If she's taking an anti-anxiety medication, this will be very short-term, usually on an "as-needed" basis.

- If her depression was very severe or if she has a strong history of previous depressions, it is possible she will need to stay on the antidepressants longer term.

SUPPORT

FIFTY-FOUR:

"I can't take anymore."

WHY YOU NEED SUPPORT, TOO

• PPD affects the whole family.

• Living with her depression will take its toll on you.

• Chances are good that her depression will deplete you of your resources. You'll be on overload for a while—increase in childcare duties, increase in household duties, decrease in sleep, increase in worry and stress—only touches the tip of the iceberg!

• Do not underestimate the impact your wife's symptoms and your extra duties will have on you.

• She needs you to take care of yourself.

FIFTY-FIVE:

"I don't need anything right now"

FIND THE TIME TO TAKE CARE OF YOURSELF

• Sometimes it seems easier to keep going the way you're going.

• Stop and think about whether you are taking care of yourself adequately:

  ✦ Are you getting enough sleep?

  ✦ Are you eating well?

  ✦ Are you getting any exercise?

  ✦ Are you overdoing anything?

  ✦ Are you exhausted?

  ✦ Are you irritable?

  ✦ Are you getting sick more often?

• Try to pay attention to how you are feeling and what you can do to take care of yourself.

- Don't put yourself on the bottom of the list of things to do. She needs you at your best right now.

FIFTY-SIX:

"I'm fine."

GIVE YOURSELF CREDIT

• She is lucky to have you by her side.

• You are working very hard right now. Every day is hard.

• Accept the fact that some days you will not be at your best.

• Try not to blame her or yourself.

• Try to work in a break now and then.

FIFTY-SEVEN:

"I know just what to do for myself"

A WORD OF CAUTION ABOUT COMFORT MEASURES

- If you are vulnerable, in any way, to addictive or self-destructive behaviors, be especially careful.

- Alcohol, cigarettes, drugs, working longer hours, staying out late . . . some of these may sound appealing at times of stress.

- None of these is a productive coping strategy. They may feel soothing in the short run, but can prove disastrous if they are your only outlets.

- If you find you are relying on support from dangerous territory, step back and approach the situation honestly. Contact a support person or therapist to get you through this.

SPECIAL
CONSIDERATIONS

FIFTY-EIGHT:

"She thinks nothing is wrong except our marriage."

HELPING YOUR WIFE GET THE HELP SHE NEEDS

- The depression will impair her ability to think clearly.

- If she is blaming you for the way she is feeling, it is quite possible that there are underlying issues related to the marriage, but this is *not* the time to work on them.

- If your wife resists treatment, you will feel isolated and extremely frustrated. If this continues, the frustration undoubtedly will lead to anger and fear.

- Her denial may be an indication that the illness is severe.

- If this is the case, it is imperative that you get help. This may mean finding a therapist for *you*, for the time being, rather than for her, so you can begin to get some perspective and guidance.

FIFTY-NINE:

*"She hasn't eaten in a couple of days and
she's not sleeping at all."*

STRATEGIES FOR INTERVENTION

- No sleep, means up all night, sleeping less than 2 hours per
  night, for a few nights in a row.

- Sleep deprivation will exacerbate everything else that's taking
  place right now.

- Taking steps to maximize her ability to sleep is one of the most
  important things you can do. This may mean:

  - Encouraging her to be evaluated for medication

  - Making plans for babysitters

  - Enlisting family members to come over and help
    while she rests

  - Taking over midnight duties.

- She has to eat. If she has no appetite, make sure she has some
  adequate intake of food that's easy to prepare and digest: yo-
  gurt, pasta, fruit. Complex carbohydrates are the best. They
  are associated with an increase in Serotonin, which will help

her feel better. How about offering a bowl of oatmeal in mid afternoon?

- She also needs to drink plenty of fluids such as water and fruit juices, especially if she is breastfeeding.

- She should avoid all refined sugars, fatty foods, junk food, alcohol, and caffeine.

SIXTY:

"She doesn't believe what her doctor is telling her."

RESISTANCE AND TREATMENT SABOTAGE

• She's scared.

• She needs reassurance.

• Ask her if she wants you to go with her. Accompany her to her appointments, whether it's her doctor, psychiatrist, or therapist. Allowing her to overindulge her dependency on you is okay for now.

• Encourage her to talk about her concerns.

• Do not yield to the enticing option of supporting her withdrawal from treatment, especially if your foremost concern is financial. It's a mistake that you definitely will pay for, in the long run.

SIXTY-ONE:

"What do I say to our parents and the rest of the family?"

DECIDE TOGETHER WHAT TO SHARE WITH OTHERS

- You and your wife are the best judges of who should know what. Decide together who will understand the nature of this information and who will be most supportive.

- Respect you or your wife's hesitation to share the details, but remember that getting support is vital.

- You can let caring friends and family know you are both struggling with this illness, but be careful to protect yourself from misguided responses, like "Oh, I never had time to be depressed!" The best response to statements that are made by people who are insensitive or misinformed is, "I'm sorry you don't understand." OR, simply, no response works in some situations, when a dialogue would just heighten your discomfort.

- Try to reflect, as honestly as possible, how much of your reluctance to talk about this is due to embarrassment or shame or fear that others won't understand. Search deep inside yourself to see if, in fact, something might be gained by letting someone you trust inside.

SIXTY-TWO:

"My four-year-old knows something is up."

TALKING WITH YOUR OLDER CHILDREN

- A child's fantasies are far worse than the reality of what's happening. Depending on his/her age, your child needs information, but not specifics.

- The best rule of thumb is to let your children know that "Mommy doesn't feel good and she's going to a doctor to get better. That's why she's crying a lot and feeling sad. She loves you very much and soon, she will be all better."

- Encourage your wife to spend time with the other children, as she feels stronger, so they can be reassured that she is still there for them.

- You should take the older children out and distract them by engaging them in a pleasurable activity so you can all enjoy some quality time together.

RECOVERY

SIXTY-THREE:

*"I thought she was getting better,
but she's still having bad days."*

THE LONG, SLOW HEALING PROCESS...

- It is possible that you will think she is getting better before *she feels she is getting better.*

- Offer bits of encouragement, but do not presume a certain level of recovery has been achieved until you *check it out with her.*

- Help her identify specific ways she is improving.

- Remind her that you understand she has a way to go until she feels like herself again – or she will think you misunderstand how bad *she still feels.*

- Remember that while she will have better days, she also will have down days in-between. These are normal and not necessarily indications of a relapse.

- Expect significant ups and downs during the recovery process.

- She may be afraid to tell you she's feeling a little better for fear you will think she's "back to normal" and expect more from her than she feels capable of doing.

- Be careful not to anticipate full recovery too soon. Acknowledge the progress and continue to support her areas of vulnerability.

- She needs to feel good for a considerable period of time before she can comfortably settle into recovery.

- Continue to take one day at a time.

SIXTY-FOUR:

"Aren't we through with this yet?"

HANGING IN THROUGH RECOVERY

- Recovery takes a long time. It will not happen as quickly as you would like it to.

- If you expect too much from her, you will sabotage her recovery.

- Get as much support as you can from others during this difficult time.

- Be encouraged by the intermittent signs of improvement, but remember to be patient and continue to protect her areas of vulnerability.

- Give yourself a great deal of credit for persevering through such difficult circumstances.

- Find ways to reward yourself and your wife.

SIXTY-FIVE:

"Now she's feeling better and I'm falling apart!"

ROLE-REVERSAL

- Do not be alarmed if you notice yourself feeling increasingly unsteady as she proceeds successfully through recovery.

- This is quite common.

- You have been carrying the extra load for a considerable amount of time.

- If you find yourself feeling more tired, angry, irritable, moody, nervous than usual . . . take note. Keep an eye on these feelings and make sure you continue (or start) taking care of *yourself* now, after all you've done for your wife and your marriage. It is more important than ever, now.

- If, at any time, you are worried about how you are feeling, do not hesitate to talk to your doctor about this.

SIXTY-SIX:

"She's feeling better . . . now what?"

TAKING CARE OF EACH OTHER AND THE MARRIAGE

- Most marriages experience considerable disruption and disturbance of balance during PPD. It is expected that this will not feel comfortable at various times.

- You may both have been exposed to sides of each other and the relationship that previously were unknown to you. This can be both unsettling and meaningful at the same time.

- Try to use what you have learned to help you stay in touch with your relationship and your understanding of how it works best.

- Remember that your marriage has just endured one of its greatest challenges.

- This is a good time to connect as a couple and resume activities that you both found pleasurable.

- Do not rule out the possibility that this experience will alter your relationship permanently. This is not necessarily a bad thing. You may both have been changed in ways that will make your marriage stronger and more meaningful.

SIXTY-SEVEN:

"Will this happen again if we have another baby?"

PLANNING FOR THE FUTURE

- Research shows us that chances are 50/50 that your wife will suffer from an episode of PPD after subsequent pregnancies. This means she is just as likely not to get it again.

- Many couples go ahead and plan for another baby after a previous episode of PPD.

- Many couples decide not to have another baby after an episode of PPD.

- This decision should be weighed carefully and should be discussed between the couple and the supervising physician. Often, this decision is determined by the severity of the illness and postpartum support that would be available.

- Couples who decide to plan another pregnancy should develop a treatment plan with the ob-gyn, pediatrician and psychiatrist or family doctor.

- This plan should include a discussion of therapy, medication, support and help at home, childcare arrangement, and breastfeeding or bottlefeeding plans. In addition, a discussion about what helped last time and what didn't help should take place.

• This more prepared you are, the more control you will have over the situation.

• Remember, no matter how prepared you are, you and your wife *may* experience another episode of PPD. In the event that this occurs, you will be better informed and have resources available, which likely will reduce PPD's impact on you as a couple, the next time around.

SIXTY-EIGHT:

"We made it though"

HOW THINGS HAVE CHANGED

- You and your wife have been through an enormous ordeal.

- Some things will be back to normal after recovery. Some things will change permanently.

- You may be confused about some of these changes. You might be pleasantly surprised by some of them.

- Or you may not notice the changes.

- Most women confess that a newfound strength has emerged within themselves and within their marriage as a direct result of the PPD crisis.

- If she is in therapy, this is a very good time to attend a session with her and discuss some of the ways this experience has affected you as a couple.

- Adjustments made during this experience can leads to striking changes in the relationship.

- This is because the events that transpired have challenged the two of you in ways that were new to both of you.

- Greater intimacy can be associated with this opportunity.

- Pay attention to what you have experienced and learned throughout this crisis, it can serve as a turning point in your relationship. It has the power to disturb the core that holds the two of you together or it can fortify and revitalize the bond hereafter.

❧

CPSIA information can be obtained at www.ICGtesting.com
Printed in the USA
LVOW06s1548021013

355119LV00001B/223/A